APPLIED ANATOMY IN CLINICAL PRACTICE

Dr Essam Abdelhakim

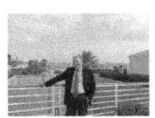

Copyright © 2024 Dr Essam Abdelhakim

All rights reserved

The characters and events portrayed in this book are fictitious. Any similarity to real persons, living or dead, is coincidental and not intended by the author.

No part of this book may be reproduced, or stored in a retrieval system, or transmitted in any form or by any means, electronic, mechanical, photocopying, recording, or otherwise, without express written permission of the publisher.

Cover design by: Art Painter
Library of Congress Control Number: 2018675309
Printed in the United States of America

CONTENTS

Title Page
Copyright
Disclosure
Introduction 1
Anatomy Relevant to Fractures 2
Anatomy in Surgeries 9
Anatomy in Imaging 15
Neuroanatomy and Its Clinical Correlates 19
Genitourinary Anatomy and Its Clinical Correlates 32
Anatomy of the Thoracic Cavity 37
Clinical Scenarios and Case Studies 41
Tips and Tricks for Applied Anatomy in Practice 62
About The Author 69

DISCLOSURE

Disclosure
This book has been created with the assistance of *Artificial Intelligence (AI) tools* and thoroughly reviewed and edited by the author to ensure clarity, relevance, and educational value.

While every effort has been made to provide accurate and up-to-date information, this content is intended solely for educational and informational purposes.

The author is a medical professional; however, the information provided in this book *is not a substitute for professional medical advice, diagnosis, or treatment.*

Readers are strongly advised to consult licensed healthcare providers or specialists for any medical concerns or conditions.

By using this book, **you acknowledge and agree** that the author shall not be held responsible or liable for any loss, damage, or harm whether physical, emotional, financial, or otherwise that may occur *as a result of the use or misuse of the information presented herein.*

INTRODUCTION

Applied anatomy bridges the gap between theoretical knowledge and practical application, making it a cornerstone of clinical practice.

Understanding anatomy in a clinical context helps healthcare professionals:

- **Diagnose Accurately:** Recognize patterns of injury or disease based on anatomical relationships. For example, identifying nerve damage in a humeral fracture by correlating symptoms with the radial nerve's path.
- **Perform Procedures Safely:** Navigate surgical interventions and minimize complications by respecting anatomical landmarks and variations. Surgeons rely on precise knowledge of structures like Calot's triangle during a cholecystectomy to prevent bile duct injuries.
- **Interpret Imaging Effectively:** Apply anatomical knowledge to identify abnormalities in radiographs, CT scans, or MRIs. This skill is essential for pinpointing fractures, tumors, or vascular anomalies.
- **Manage Emergencies:** Quick anatomical reasoning is critical in life-threatening scenarios such as airway obstruction or spinal cord injuries.

ANATOMY RELEVANT TO FRACTURES

Upper Limb Fractures

Clavicle: Mechanism of Injury and Structures at Risk

The clavicle, commonly fractured in falls or direct trauma, acts as a strut between the sternum and scapula.

Key clinical considerations include:

- **Mechanism of Injury:** Typically caused by a fall onto the shoulder or outstretched hand.
- **Structures at Risk:** The brachial plexus and subclavian vessels lie posterior to the clavicle and may be injured in high-energy fractures.
- **Clinical Features:** Pain, deformity, and potential neurovascular compromise.

Humerus: Surgical Neck And Radial Nerve Injury

Fractures of the surgical neck are prevalent in older adults following low-energy falls.

- **Radial Nerve:** Courses in the spiral groove of the humerus; injury leads to wrist drop and sensory loss in the dorsal hand.
- **Management:** Includes conservative treatment or surgical fixation depending on displacement and nerve involvement.

Forearm

Monteggia And Galeazzi Fractures

Monteggia Fractures:

- **Definition**: Fractures of the proximal third of the ulna with dislocation of the radial head at the elbow.
- **Mechanism of Injury**: Typically caused by a fall on an outstretched hand with the forearm in pronation.
- **Structures at Risk**:
    - **Radial Nerve**: Due to its proximity to the radial head.
    - **Interosseous Membrane**: Essential for forearm stability.

Galeazzi Fractures:

- **Definition**: Fractures of the distal third of the radius with dislocation or subluxation of the distal radioulnar joint (DRUJ).
- **Mechanism of Injury**: Often results from direct trauma to the wrist or a fall on an outstretched hand.
- **Structures at Risk**:
    - **Ulnar Nerve**: Due to its proximity to the DRUJ.
    - **Triangular Fibrocartilage Complex (TFCC)**: Critical for DRUJ stability.

Wrist

Scaphoid And Colles' Fractures

Scaphoid Fractures:

- **Definition**: Fractures of the scaphoid bone, the most commonly injured carpal bone.
- **Mechanism of Injury**: Caused by a fall on an outstretched hand with wrist extension.
- **Structures at Risk**:
    - **Radial Artery**: Supplies the proximal pole, putting it at risk for avascular necrosis if the fracture disrupts blood flow.

Colles' Fractures:

- **Definition**: Fractures of the distal radius with dorsal angulation, commonly seen in older adults with osteoporosis.
- **Mechanism of Injury**: Result of a fall on an outstretched hand.
- **Structures at Risk**:
    - **Median Nerve**: At risk for compression in cases of severe angulation or swelling.
    - **Flexor Tendons**: May be compromised by sharp fracture edges.

Lower Limb Fractures

Hip: Femoral Neck Fractures And Avascular Necrosis

Femoral Neck Fractures:

- **Definition**: Fractures occurring within the capsule of the hip joint.
- **Mechanism of Injury**: Commonly due to low-energy falls in the elderly or high-energy trauma in younger individuals.
- **Structures at Risk**:
    - **Medial Femoral Circumflex Artery**: Primary blood supply to the femoral head, increasing the risk of avascular necrosis.

Avascular Necrosis (Avn):

- **Definition**: Death of bone tissue due to disrupted blood supply.
- **Clinical Relevance**: A common complication of femoral neck fractures.
- **Key Symptoms**: Groin pain and reduced range of motion.

Tibia: Compartment Syndrome And Nerve Involvement

Compartment Syndrome:

- **Definition**: Increased pressure within a closed fascial

compartment, leading to ischemia and tissue damage.
- **Mechanism of Injury**: Often associated with tibial fractures due to swelling or bleeding within the compartments.
- **Structures at Risk**:
  - **Deep Peroneal Nerve**: Involved in dorsiflexion; damage leads to foot drop.
  - **Tibial Artery**: Essential for lower leg perfusion.

Ankle: Lateral Malleolus And Syndesmotic Injuries

Lateral Malleolus Fractures:

- **Definition**: Fractures of the distal fibula.
- **Mechanism of Injury**: Caused by twisting or rolling of the ankle.
- **Structures at Risk**:
  - **Superficial Peroneal Nerve**: Located near the distal fibula.

Syndesmotic Injuries:

- **Definition**: Injuries to the ligaments connecting the tibia and fibula above the ankle joint.
- **Mechanism of Injury**: High-energy rotational injuries.
- **Structures at Risk**:
  - **Interosseous Ligament**: Critical for maintaining tibiofibular stability.

Spine Fractures

Cervical Spine: Jefferson And Hangman Fractures

Jefferson Fractures:

- **Definition**: Burst fractures of the C1 vertebra (atlas).
- **Mechanism of Injury**: Axial loading, such as a heavy object falling on the head.
- **Structures at Risk**:
  - **Vertebral Arteries**: Due to their passage through the transverse foramen of C1.

Hangman Fractures:

- **Definition**: Fractures of the pars interarticularis of the C2 vertebra (axis).
- **Mechanism of Injury**: Hyperextension injuries, such as in motor vehicle accidents.
- **Structures at Risk**:
  - **Spinal Cord**: At risk for compression in severe cases.

Thoracolumbar Spine: Burst And Chance Fractures

Burst Fractures:

- **Definition**: Fractures involving compression and bursting of a vertebral body.
- **Mechanism of Injury**: High-energy axial loading.
- **Structures at Risk**:
  - **Spinal Cord and Nerve Roots**: Potentially

compressed by bone fragments.

Chance Fractures:

- **Definition**: Horizontal fractures through the vertebral body and posterior elements.
- **Mechanism of Injury**: Flexion-distraction injuries, often from seatbelt trauma.
- **Structures at Risk**:
    - **Posterior Ligaments**: Often disrupted.
    - **Spinal Cord**: Risk of severe neurological compromise.

ANATOMY IN SURGERIES

General Principles Of Surgical Anatomy

Understanding Anatomical Variations

- **Definition**: Anatomical variations are deviations from typical anatomical structures that are not pathological.
- **Importance**: Recognizing variations can prevent complications, especially in surgeries near critical structures like nerves, vessels, or ducts.
- **Examples**:
    - Accessory renal arteries during nephrectomy.
    - Variations in bile duct anatomy during cholecystectomy.

Safe Dissection Techniques

- **Key Points**:
    - Use blunt dissection near vital structures to minimize accidental injury.
    - Maintain clear visualization of the surgical field.
    - Employ hemostatic techniques to reduce bleeding and improve visibility.

Identification Of Danger Zones

- **Definition**: Regions with a high density of vital structures or increased risk of injury during surgery.
- **Examples**:
  - **Calot's Triangle** during cholecystectomy: Risk of bile duct or cystic artery injury.
  - **Inguinal Canal** during hernia repairs: Risk of ilioinguinal nerve damage.
  - **Tracheoesophageal Groove** during thyroidectomy: Risk of recurrent laryngeal nerve injury.

Common Surgical Procedures

Appendectomy: Location Of The Appendix And Surrounding Structures

- **Anatomical Features**:
  - The appendix is typically located in the right lower quadrant at the junction of the taeniae coli.
  - Variations include retrocecal, pelvic, subcecal, or pre-ileal positions.
- **Surrounding Structures**:
  - **Cecum and Terminal Ileum**: Avoid damage during mobilization.
  - **Iliac Vessels**: Important to identify and preserve during dissection.

Cholecystectomy: Calot's Triangle And Risk Of Bile Duct Injury

- **Calot's Triangle**:

- Bounded by the cystic duct, common hepatic duct, and inferior surface of the liver.
- Key landmark for identifying the cystic artery and cystic duct.
- **Complications**:
  - Variations in cystic artery anatomy can increase the risk of bile duct injury.
  - The right hepatic duct or artery may traverse the triangle, requiring meticulous dissection.

Hernia Repairs: Inguinal Canal Anatomy And Variants

- **Anatomy of the Inguinal Canal**:
  - Contains the spermatic cord (males) or round ligament (females).
  - The ilioinguinal nerve courses nearby, at risk during dissection.
- **Types of Hernias**:
  - **Direct Hernias**: Occur medial to the inferior epigastric vessels through Hesselbach's triangle.
  - **Indirect Hernias**: Occur lateral to the inferior epigastric vessels and follow the inguinal canal.

Thyroidectomy: Recurrent Laryngeal Nerve And Parathyroid Glands

- **Recurrent Laryngeal Nerve**:
  - Runs in the tracheoesophageal groove.
  - Injury can lead to vocal cord paralysis and

hoarseness.
- **Parathyroid Glands:**
    - Typically located posterior to the thyroid gland.
    - Inadvertent removal can cause hypocalcemia; preserving their blood supply is crucial.

Orthopedic Surgeries

Total Hip Replacement: Acetabulum And Femoral Components

- **Acetabular Component**:
    - Proper positioning ensures stability and minimizes dislocations.
    - Over- or under-coverage can affect joint longevity.
- **Femoral Component**:
    - Alignment with the medullary canal optimizes load distribution and reduces stress on the prosthesis.

Acl Reconstruction: Anatomical Grafts And Landmarks

- **Anterior Cruciate Ligament (ACL)**:
    - Originates from the intercondylar notch of the femur.
    - Inserts on the tibial plateau.
- **Graft Placement**:
    - Should replicate native ligament orientation to restore knee stability.
    - Incorrect placement can lead to persistent instability or limited range of motion.

Rotator Cuff Repairs: Anatomy Of The Shoulder Joint

- **Rotator Cuff**:
    - Composed of four muscles: supraspinatus, infraspinatus, teres minor, and subscapularis.
    - Stabilizes the shoulder joint and facilitates movement.
- **Surgical Considerations**:
    - Repairs often involve reattaching torn tendons to the greater tuberosity of the humerus.
    - Preservation of the subacromial space reduces impingement risk.

ANATOMY IN IMAGING

Radiographic Anatomy: Key Landmarks On X-Rays

Chest: Heart Borders And Lung Lobes

- **Heart Borders**:
    - **Right Border**: Formed by the right atrium.
    - **Left Border**: Composed of the left ventricle and part of the left atrium.
    - **Inferior Border**: Formed by the right ventricle.
    - **Clinical Importance**: Enlarged borders can indicate pathologies like cardiomegaly or pericardial effusion.
- **Lung Lobes**:
    - Right lung has three lobes (upper, middle, lower) and is divided by the horizontal and oblique fissures.
    - Left lung has two lobes (upper and lower) separated by the oblique fissure.
    - **Clinical Importance**: Identifying lobar consolidations or pneumothorax.

Abdomen: Gas Patterns And Organ Shadows

- **Gas Patterns**:
    - Stomach bubble under the left diaphragm.

- Intestinal gas in loops of the small and large bowel.
- **Clinical Importance**: Free air under the diaphragm suggests perforation.
- **Organ Shadows**:
  - **Liver**: Right upper quadrant shadow.
  - **Spleen**: Left upper quadrant shadow.
  - **Clinical Importance**: Displacement may indicate masses or trauma.

Skeletal: Fracture Identification And Joint Alignment

- **Fracture Identification**:
  - Look for cortical breaks, step-offs, or displacement.
  - **Common Sites**: Long bones, vertebrae, and pelvis.
- **Joint Alignment**:
  - Assess for congruity of joint spaces.
  - **Clinical Importance**: Dislocations and subluxations.

Cross-Sectional Imaging: Ct And Mri Correlates

Head And Neck: Sinuses, Brain, And Skull Base

- **Sinuses**:
  - Maxillary, frontal, ethmoid, and sphenoid sinuses are visible on CT.
  - **Clinical Importance**: Sinusitis or fractures

from trauma.
- **Brain:**
  - Key landmarks include the ventricles, basal ganglia, and cerebral cortex.
  - **Clinical Importance**: Hemorrhages, strokes, or tumors.
- **Skull Base:**
  - Contains foramina for cranial nerves and vessels.
  - **Clinical Importance**: Skull base fractures affecting cranial nerves.

Spine: Disc Herniations And Nerve Roots

- **Disc Herniations:**
  - Seen as bulging or extrusion of the intervertebral disc on MRI.
  - **Clinical Importance**: Compresses nerve roots causing radiculopathy.
- **Nerve Roots:**
  - Best visualized in the axial and sagittal planes.
  - **Clinical Importance**: Impingement or inflammation causing pain and weakness.

Joints: Labral Tears and Ligament Injuries

- **Labral Tears:**
  - Common in the shoulder (glenoid labrum) and hip (acetabular labrum).
  - **MRI Findings**: Contrast leakage or irregularity in labral contour.
  - **Clinical Importance**: Associated with instability or pain.

- **Ligament Injuries**:
    - ACL, PCL, and other ligament tears are best seen on MRI.
    - **Clinical Importance**: Instability or restricted joint function.

NEUROANATOMY AND ITS CLINICAL CORRELATES

Brain Anatomy

Lobes Of The Brain And Their Functions

- **Frontal Lobe**:
    - Functions: Executive functions, decision-making, motor control, and speech production (Broca's area).
    - Clinical Correlates: Lesions can cause personality changes, motor deficits, or expressive aphasia.
- **Parietal Lobe**:
    - Functions: Sensory processing, spatial awareness, and proprioception.
    - Clinical Correlates: Damage may result in sensory loss or neglect syndrome.
- **Temporal Lobe**:
    - Functions: Hearing, memory, and understanding language (Wernicke's area).
    - Clinical Correlates: Lesions can cause receptive aphasia or memory disturbances.
- **Occipital Lobe**:
    - Functions: Visual processing and interpretation.

- Clinical Correlates: Lesions may lead to visual field defects or cortical blindness.

Basal Ganglia: Disorders And Pathways

- **Anatomy**:
  - Comprises the caudate nucleus, putamen, globus pallidus, subthalamic nucleus, and substantia nigra.
  - Connected by complex loops to the cortex and thalamus.
- **Functions**:
  - Regulates motor control, movement initiation, and procedural learning.
- **Clinical Correlates**:
  - Parkinson's Disease: Due to degeneration of dopaminergic neurons in the substantia nigra.
  - Huntington's Disease: Caused by atrophy of the caudate nucleus, leading to chorea and dementia.
  - Hemiballismus: Lesion in the subthalamic nucleus causing involuntary flinging movements.

Cerebellum: Ataxia And Coordination Issues

- **Anatomy**:
  - Divided into anterior, posterior, and flocculonodular lobes.
  - Connected to the brainstem via superior, middle, and inferior peduncles.
- **Functions**:

- Coordinates voluntary movements, balance, and posture.
- **Clinical Correlates**:
  - Lesions cause ataxia, dysmetria, intention tremor, and nystagmus.
  - Midline lesions (vermis) affect trunk stability, while lateral lesions affect limb coordination.

Cranial Nerves

Overview And Functions

- **Cranial Nerves I–XII**:
    - Olfactory (I): Smell.
    - Optic (II): Vision.
    - Oculomotor (III), Trochlear (IV), and Abducens (VI): Eye movements.
    - Trigeminal (V): Facial sensation and mastication.
    - Facial (VII): Facial expression and taste (anterior 2/3 of the tongue).
    - Vestibulocochlear (VIII): Hearing and balance.
    - Glossopharyngeal (IX) and Vagus (X): Taste, swallowing, and autonomic functions.
    - Accessory (XI): Shoulder and neck movement.
    - Hypoglossal (XII): Tongue movement.

Common Lesions: Clinical Presentation And Localization

- **Optic Nerve (II)**: Lesions cause vision loss or visual field defects (e.g., bitemporal hemianopia in chiasmal lesions).
- **Facial Nerve (VII)**: Bell's palsy causes unilateral facial paralysis.

- **Trigeminal Nerve (V)**: Lesions lead to facial pain (trigeminal neuralgia) or loss of sensation.
- **Oculomotor Nerve (III)**: Ptosis, eye deviation down and out, and pupil dilation.

Case Studies

- **Bell's Palsy:**
    - Sudden onset of unilateral facial weakness.
    - Often associated with viral infections.
    - Resolves spontaneously in most cases.
- **Trigeminal Neuralgia:**
    - Severe, episodic facial pain triggered by light touch.
    - Treated with carbamazepine or surgical decompression.
- **Optic Neuritis:**
    - Painful vision loss often associated with multiple sclerosis.
    - Managed with corticosteroids.

Spinal Cord

Anatomy And Segmental Levels

- **Structure:**
    - Extends from the medulla oblongata to the conus medullaris (L1–L2).
    - Divided into cervical, thoracic, lumbar, sacral, and coccygeal segments.
- **Landmarks:**

- C5–T1: Brachial plexus.
- L2–S3: Lumbosacral plexus.
- Reflex arcs (e.g., patellar reflex at L3–L4).

Common Syndromes

- **Brown-Séquard Syndrome**:
    - Hemisection of the spinal cord.
    - Ipsilateral motor loss and proprioception with contralateral pain/temperature loss.
- **Central Cord Syndrome**:
    - Affects cervical spinal cord, causing greater motor impairment in upper limbs than lower limbs.
    - Commonly seen in hyperextension injuries.
- **Anterior Cord Syndrome**:
    - Loss of motor function and pain/temperature sensation below the lesion.
    - Preserved dorsal column functions (proprioception and vibration).

Cranial Nerve Lesions

Olfactory Nerve (Cn I): Loss Of Smell In Head Trauma

The olfactory nerve is responsible for the sense of smell and is often affected in cases of head trauma. The nerve fibers pass through the cribriform plate of the ethmoid bone, making them vulnerable to shearing injuries during rapid deceleration or blunt force trauma.

- **Clinical Presentation**: Loss of smell (anosmia) without nasal congestion or sinus disease.
- **Diagnosis**: History and physical examination, including testing each nostril separately for the ability to identify familiar odors.
- **Clinical Correlation**: Anosmia may also result from neurodegenerative disorders such as Parkinson's or Alzheimer's disease.

Optic Nerve (Cn Ii): Visual Field Defects In Optic Neuritis

The optic nerve transmits visual information from the retina to the brain. Optic neuritis, often associated with multiple sclerosis, leads to inflammation and demyelination.

- **Clinical Presentation**: Sudden vision loss, pain with eye movement, and decreased color vision (dyschromatopsia).
- **Visual Field Defects**: Central scotoma is a common finding.
- **Diagnosis**: Fundoscopy may reveal optic disc swelling (papillitis), and MRI often shows enhancement of the optic nerve.
- **Treatment**: Corticosteroids to reduce inflammation and manage symptoms.

Oculomotor, Trochlear, And Abducens Nerves (Cn Iii, Iv, Vi): Eye Movement Disorders

These cranial nerves control the muscles responsible for eye movements.

- **CN III (Oculomotor)**: Innervates most extraocular muscles, except the lateral rectus and superior oblique.

Lesions result in ptosis, "down and out" eye position, and pupil dilation.
- **CN IV (Trochlear)**: Innervates the superior oblique muscle. Lesions cause difficulty looking down and in, often resulting in vertical diplopia.
- **CN VI (Abducens)**: Innervates the lateral rectus muscle. Lesions cause horizontal diplopia and inability to abduct the eye.
- **Common Causes**: Microvascular ischemia (diabetes, hypertension), trauma, and compressive lesions such as aneurysms.

Facial Nerve (Cn Vii): Facial Paralysis And Synkinesis

The facial nerve controls facial expressions, taste sensation on the anterior two-thirds of the tongue, and lacrimal and salivary glands.

- **Bell's Palsy**: Acute, idiopathic facial nerve paralysis, often preceded by viral infection.
  - **Clinical Features**: Inability to close the eye, drooping mouth, loss of nasolabial fold, and hyperacusis.
  - **Treatment**: Corticosteroids and antivirals in some cases.
- **Synkinesis**: Aberrant regeneration of the facial nerve, leading to simultaneous contraction of different facial muscles.
- **Differential Diagnosis**: Stroke (upper motor neuron lesions spare the forehead).

Glossopharyngeal And Vagus Nerves (Cn Ix, X): Dysphagia And Voice Changes

The glossopharyngeal and vagus nerves play a role in swallowing, phonation, and sensation in the throat.

- **CN IX (Glossopharyngeal)**: Lesions result in impaired gag reflex, loss of taste on the posterior third of the tongue, and difficulty swallowing.
- **CN X (Vagus)**: Lesions lead to hoarseness, uvula deviation away from the side of the lesion, and impaired swallowing.
- **Common Causes**: Surgery (e.g., carotid endarterectomy), tumors, and stroke.
- **Diagnosis**: Observation of uvula position, gag reflex testing, and laryngoscopy.

Accessory Nerve (Cn Xi): Shoulder Weakness

The accessory nerve innervates the sternocleidomastoid and trapezius muscles.
- **Clinical Presentation**: Weakness in shrugging the shoulder (trapezius) and difficulty turning the head to the opposite side (sternocleidomastoid).
- **Common Causes**: Neck surgery, trauma, and compression.
- **Diagnosis**: Electromyography (EMG) and clinical examination.

Hypoglossal Nerve (Cn Xii): Tongue Deviation

The hypoglossal nerve controls tongue movements.
- **Clinical Presentation**: Tongue deviation toward the side of the lesion, atrophy, and fasciculations on the affected side.
- **Common Causes**: Tumors, stroke, or neck surgery.
- **Diagnosis**: Observation during tongue protrusion and assessment of speech and swallowing difficulties.

Spinal Cord Syndromes

Anatomy Of The Spinal Cord

The spinal cord extends from the medulla oblongata to the level of the L1-L2 vertebrae in adults. It is organized into cervical, thoracic, lumbar, sacral, and coccygeal segments. Gray matter (neuronal cell bodies) is centrally located, surrounded by white matter (ascending and descending tracts). The spinal cord is supplied by the anterior spinal artery and paired posterior spinal arteries.

Upper Motor Neuron vs. Lower Motor Neuron Lesions

- **Upper Motor Neuron (UMN) Lesions:** Affect the motor cortex or corticospinal tracts, leading to spasticity, hyperreflexia, and the Babinski sign.
- **Lower Motor Neuron (LMN) Lesions:** Affect the anterior horn cells or peripheral nerves, resulting in flaccidity, hyporeflexia, and muscle atrophy.

Clinical Syndromes

Complete Cord Transection: Motor And Sensory Loss

Complete transection of the spinal cord results in:
- **Motor Loss:** Paralysis below the level of the lesion (tetraplegia or paraplegia depending on the level).
- **Sensory Loss:** Complete loss of all modalities below the lesion.
- **Autonomic Dysfunction:** Loss of bowel, bladder, and sexual function. Emergency management includes spinal immobilization and surgical decompression.

Hemicord Lesion (Brown-Séquard Syndrome): Asymmetric Findings

A hemicord lesion causes:
- **Ipsilateral:** Weakness and loss of proprioception/vibration sense (corticospinal and dorsal column involvement).
- **Contralateral:** Loss of pain and temperature sensation (spinothalamic tract involvement). This pattern often arises from penetrating trauma or spinal tumors.

Central Cord Syndrome: Upper Limb Predominance

This syndrome typically occurs with cervical spinal cord injuries and **results in:**
- Weakness greater in the upper limbs than lower limbs.
- Variable sensory loss.
- Preservation of sacral sensation. Common causes include hyperextension injuries and syringomyelia.

Cauda Equina Syndrome: Saddle Anesthesia And Bladder Dysfunction

Compression of the cauda equina (L2-S5 nerve roots) results in:
- **Sensory:** Saddle anesthesia.
- **Motor:** Asymmetric lower limb weakness.
- **Autonomic:** Bowel and bladder dysfunction. This is a surgical emergency requiring prompt decompression to prevent permanent deficits.

GENITOURINARY ANATOMY AND ITS CLINICAL CORRELATES

Anatomy Of The Kidneys

- **Location:** The kidneys are retroperitoneal organs located at the level of T12–L3 vertebrae. The right kidney is slightly lower due to the liver.
- **Surrounding Structures:** Each kidney is surrounded by the renal fascia, perirenal fat, and pararenal fat, which provide cushioning and protection.
- **Clinical Correlates:**
    - **Renal Trauma:** The kidneys are vulnerable to blunt and penetrating injuries. The proximity to the 12th rib increases the risk of fractures causing renal injury.
    - **Hydronephrosis:** Obstruction in the urinary tract, such as from kidney stones, can cause dilation of the renal pelvis and calyces.

Ureters

- **Course:** Ureters are muscular tubes that transport urine from the kidneys to the bladder. They descend retroperitoneally, crossing the iliac vessels and entering the bladder obliquely.
- **Clinical Correlates:**

- **Ureteric Stones:** Common sites of obstruction include the pelviureteric junction, crossing of the iliac vessels, and the vesicoureteric junction. Pain radiates to the flank or groin depending on the level of obstruction.
- **Surgical Injury:** The ureters are at risk during pelvic surgeries, such as hysterectomy, due to their close relationship with the uterine arteries.

Urinary Bladder

- **Anatomy:** The bladder is a hollow organ located in the pelvis, posterior to the pubic symphysis. It has a trigone formed by the ureteral openings and the internal urethral orifice.
- **Clinical Correlates:**
  - **Bladder Outlet Obstruction:** Common causes include benign prostatic hyperplasia (BPH) and bladder neck stenosis, leading to urinary retention.
  - **Trauma:** Rupture of the bladder can occur in pelvic fractures, particularly if it is distended at the time of injury.

Male Reproductive Anatomy

- **Prostate:** The prostate gland surrounds the urethra and contributes to seminal fluid production.
  - **Clinical Correlates:**
    - **Prostate Cancer:** Often arises in the peripheral zone and can cause obstructive urinary symptoms or be

detected as an asymptomatic mass.
- **BPH:** Enlargement of the transition zone leads to compression of the urethra and obstructive voiding symptoms.

- **Testes and Scrotum:**
    - The testes are located within the scrotum and produce sperm and testosterone.
    - **Clinical Correlates:**
        - **Testicular Torsion:** Twisting of the spermatic cord compromises blood supply, requiring urgent surgical intervention.
        - **Hydrocele:** Accumulation of fluid around the testes can result from trauma or infection.

Female Reproductive Anatomy

- **Uterus:**
    - A pear-shaped organ located in the pelvis between the bladder and rectum.
    - **Clinical Correlates:**
        - **Uterine Prolapse:** Weakening of pelvic support structures can lead to descent of the uterus into the vaginal canal.
        - **Endometriosis:** Presence of endometrial tissue outside the uterus causes pelvic pain and infertility.
- **Ovaries and Fallopian Tubes:**
    - The ovaries produce oocytes and hormones,

APPLIED ANATOMY IN CLINICAL PRACTICE

while the fallopian tubes facilitate fertilization.
- **Clinical Correlates:**
  - **Ectopic Pregnancy:** Implantation of a fertilized egg in the fallopian tube is a surgical emergency due to risk of rupture.
  - **Ovarian Torsion:** Twisting of the ovary compromises blood supply and causes acute pelvic pain.

Pelvic Floor

- **Muscles:** Includes the levator ani and coccygeus, which support pelvic organs.
- **Clinical Correlates:**
  - **Pelvic Floor Dysfunction:** Weakness or injury can lead to urinary incontinence or pelvic organ prolapse.
  - **Rectocele and Cystocele:** Protrusion of the rectum or bladder into the vaginal wall, respectively, can occur following childbirth or chronic straining.

Vasculature

- **Renal Arteries and Veins:** The renal arteries arise from the abdominal aorta, while the renal veins drain into the inferior vena cava.
  - **Clinical Correlates:**
    - **Renal Artery Stenosis:** Narrowing of the renal artery can lead to hypertension and ischemic

nephropathy.
- **Nutcracker Syndrome:** Compression of the left renal vein between the aorta and superior mesenteric artery causes hematuria and flank pain.

Nerves

- **Sympathetic and Parasympathetic Supply:**
  - Sympathetic fibers originate from T10–L2, while parasympathetic fibers arise from the sacral plexus.
  - **Clinical Correlates:**
    - **Neurogenic Bladder:** Disruption of nerve supply due to spinal cord injury results in loss of bladder control.
    - **Referred Pain:** Ureteric colic pain may refer to the flank, groin, or genitals depending on the level of the obstruction.

ANATOMY OF THE THORACIC CAVITY

The thoracic cavity houses vital organs including the heart, lungs, and great vessels, as well as critical structures such as the esophagus and thoracic duct. It is divided into three compartments: the mediastinum, and two pleural cavities.

Mediastinum

- **Anatomy:** The mediastinum is divided into anterior, middle, posterior, and superior compartments, each containing specific structures:
    - **Anterior Mediastinum:** Contains thymic remnants, lymph nodes, and fat.
    - **Middle Mediastinum:** Houses the heart, pericardium, ascending aorta, pulmonary arteries, and veins.
    - **Posterior Mediastinum:** Contains the descending aorta, esophagus, thoracic duct, and sympathetic trunks.
    - **Superior Mediastinum:** Includes the great vessels (aortic arch, brachiocephalic veins), trachea, and esophagus.
- **Clinical Correlation:**
    - **Mediastinal Masses:** Symptoms depend on the location and structures compressed (e.g., dyspnea, dysphagia).

- **Cardiac Tamponade:** Accumulation of fluid in the pericardium can compress the heart, requiring emergency pericardiocentesis.

Heart Anatomy

- **Anatomy:** The heart has four chambers (right atrium, right ventricle, left atrium, left ventricle) and is supplied by coronary arteries. Key valves include the tricuspid, pulmonary, mitral, and aortic valves.
- **Clinical Correlation:**
  - **Coronary Artery Disease (CAD):** Blockages in the coronary arteries lead to myocardial ischemia and infarction.
  - **Valve Pathologies:** Conditions like mitral regurgitation or aortic stenosis can significantly impact cardiac output.

Pulmonary Anatomy

- **Anatomy:** The lungs are divided into lobes (three on the right, two on the left) and are supplied by the bronchial and pulmonary arteries. Gas exchange occurs in the alveoli.
- **Clinical Correlation:**
  - **Pneumothorax:** Air in the pleural cavity collapses the lung, requiring chest tube placement.
  - **Pulmonary Embolism (PE):** Blockage of a pulmonary artery, often by a thrombus, can cause hypoxia and require anticoagulation.

Great Vessels

- **Anatomy:** The great vessels include the aorta, pulmonary arteries and veins, superior and inferior vena cava, and their major branches.
- **Clinical Correlation:**
    - **Aortic Dissection:** A tear in the aortic wall leads to a life-threatening condition requiring immediate intervention.
    - **Superior Vena Cava Syndrome (SVCS):** Compression of the SVC causes facial swelling and distended neck veins.

Thoracic Wall And Rib Cage

- **Anatomy:** The thoracic wall includes ribs, intercostal muscles, and the sternum. The neurovascular bundle (intercostal nerve, artery, and vein) lies beneath each rib.
- **Clinical Correlation:**
    - **Rib Fractures:** Can cause pain, impaired ventilation, and puncture underlying organs.
    - **Thoracentesis:** Performed above the rib to avoid damaging the neurovascular bundle.

Diaphragm

- **Anatomy:** The diaphragm separates the thoracic and abdominal cavities and is innervated by the phrenic nerve (C3, C4, C5).
- **Clinical Correlation:**
    - **Diaphragmatic Paralysis:** Injury to the phrenic nerve results in impaired ventilation.
    - **Hiatal Hernia:** Protrusion of the stomach through the diaphragm can cause reflux

symptoms.

Esophagus

- **Anatomy:** The esophagus passes through the thoracic cavity and enters the abdomen via the esophageal hiatus in the diaphragm.
- **Clinical Correlation:**
    - **Esophageal Perforation:** Often due to trauma or Boerhaave syndrome; requires emergency intervention.
    - **GERD:** Weakness in the lower esophageal sphincter can cause acid reflux.

Sympathetic Chain And Thoracic Duct

- **Anatomy:** The sympathetic chain runs along the posterior thoracic wall, and the thoracic duct is the main lymphatic vessel.
- **Clinical Correlation:**
    - **Horner Syndrome:** Damage to the sympathetic chain results in ptosis, miosis, and anhidrosis.
    - **Chylothorax:** Leakage of lymphatic fluid into the pleural cavity can occur after thoracic surgery or trauma.

CLINICAL SCENARIOS AND CASE STUDIES

Case 1: Radial Nerve Injury After Midshaft Humerus Fracture

- **Presentation:** A 35-year-old male presents after a fall onto an outstretched arm. Radiographs confirm a midshaft humerus fracture. The patient reports weakness in wrist extension and numbness over the dorsum of the hand.
- **Anatomy Involved:** The radial nerve runs in the spiral groove of the humerus and is susceptible to injury with midshaft fractures.
- **Clinical Correlates:**
  - Wrist drop due to loss of wrist extensors.
  - Sensory loss over the dorsal hand and lateral thumb.
- **Management:**
  - Initial management includes fracture stabilization and observation for nerve recovery.
  - Surgical exploration if no improvement in nerve function within 3-6 months.

Case 2: Biliary Leak Following Laparoscopic Cholecystectomy

- **Presentation:** A 50-year-old female presents with abdominal pain and fever 3 days post-laparoscopic cholecystectomy. Imaging reveals fluid collection near the liver.
- **Anatomy Involved:** The biliary tree includes the cystic duct, common bile duct, and hepatic ducts. Injury to these structures can cause bile leakage.
- **Clinical Correlates:**
    - Symptoms include right upper quadrant pain, jaundice, and fever.
    - Diagnosis confirmed by imaging (e.g., HIDA scan, MRCP).
- **Management:**
    - Percutaneous drainage of bile collection.
    - ERCP with stent placement to divert bile flow.

Case 3: Optic Neuritis In Multiple Sclerosis

- **Presentation:** A 29-year-old female reports sudden vision loss in one eye, pain with eye movement, and reduced color vision. Fundoscopy shows optic disc swelling.
- **Anatomy Involved:** The optic nerve transmits visual signals to the brain and is affected by demyelination in multiple sclerosis.
- **Clinical Correlates:**
    - Visual field defects, reduced acuity, and pain with movement.
    - Often the first manifestation of multiple sclerosis.
- **Management:**
    - High-dose intravenous corticosteroids.
    - Referral to neurology for disease-modifying therapy.

Case 4: Anterior Cord Syndrome After Thoracic Spine Fracture

- **Presentation:** A 40-year-old male falls from a height and sustains a thoracic spine fracture. He experiences loss of motor function and pain sensation below the lesion but retains proprioception.
- **Anatomy Involved:** The anterior spinal cord houses motor tracts (corticospinal) and pain/temperature pathways (spinothalamic).
- **Clinical Correlates:**
    - Loss of motor and pain/temperature sensation.
    - Preservation of dorsal column functions (proprioception, vibration).
- **Management:**
    - Immediate spinal immobilization.
    - Surgical decompression if indicated.

Case 5: Recurrent Inguinal Hernia Repair And Nerve Entrapment

- **Presentation:** A 60-year-old male presents with chronic groin pain after recurrent inguinal hernia repair. The pain worsens with movement and is localized to the groin.
- **Anatomy Involved:** The ilioinguinal, iliohypogastric, and genitofemoral nerves are at risk during inguinal hernia repair.
- **Clinical Correlates:**
    - Nerve entrapment leads to chronic neuropathic pain.
    - Diagnosis is clinical but may be supported by nerve blocks.
- **Management:**
    - Conservative measures: analgesics, physical therapy.
    - Surgical nerve release or neurectomy for refractory cases.

Case 6: Ulnar Nerve Entrapment At The Elbow

- **Presentation:** A 45-year-old carpenter complains of numbness and tingling in the ring and little fingers, with hand weakness, particularly in grip strength. Symptoms are aggravated by prolonged elbow flexion.
- **Anatomy Involved:** The ulnar nerve passes through the cubital tunnel at the elbow and is prone to compression.
- **Clinical Correlates:**
    - Sensory loss in the medial hand.
    - Weakness of intrinsic hand muscles (e.g., interossei, hypothenar muscles).
    - Positive Tinel's sign at the elbow.
- **Management:**
    - Activity modification and elbow splinting.
    - Surgical decompression if symptoms persist or worsen.

Case 7: Femoral Nerve Injury After Pelvic Fracture

- **Presentation:** A 30-year-old male involved in a motorcycle accident sustains a pelvic fracture. He reports difficulty walking and numbness in the anterior thigh and medial calf.
- **Anatomy Involved:** The femoral nerve arises from the lumbar plexus and is vulnerable to injury in pelvic trauma.
- **Clinical Correlates:**
    - Weakness in knee extension and hip flexion.
    - Reduced patellar reflex.
    - Sensory loss over the anterior thigh and medial lower leg.
- **Management:**
    - Physical therapy for strength recovery.
    - Surgical intervention for fracture stabilization.

Case 8: Pneumothorax After Central Venous Catheter Placement

- **Presentation:** A 65-year-old male undergoing central venous catheter placement suddenly develops shortness of breath and pleuritic chest pain. Chest X-ray reveals a collapsed lung.
- **Anatomy Involved:** The apex of the lung lies near the subclavian vein, making it susceptible to puncture during catheterization.
- **Clinical Correlates:**
    - Decreased breath sounds on the affected side.
    - Tracheal deviation in tension pneumothorax.
    - Diagnosis confirmed by imaging.
- **Management:**
    - Immediate needle decompression for tension pneumothorax.
    - Chest tube insertion to re-expand the lung.

Case 9: Sciatic Nerve Injury After Hip Replacement

- **Presentation:** A 70-year-old female reports foot drop and numbness in the posterior leg following total hip arthroplasty. Examination reveals weakness in ankle dorsiflexion and eversion.
- **Anatomy Involved:** The sciatic nerve runs posteriorly near the hip joint and can be injured during surgical procedures.
- **Clinical Correlates:**
- **Clinical Correlates:**
    - Foot drop due to peroneal nerve involvement.
    - Sensory loss in the posterior leg and sole of the foot.
- **Management:**
    - Physiotherapy and ankle-foot orthosis for functional support.
    - Nerve conduction studies to assess recovery.

Case 10: Median Nerve Injury In Carpal Tunnel Syndrome

- **Presentation:** A 55-year-old office worker complains of nocturnal hand pain and numbness affecting the thumb, index, and middle fingers. Symptoms improve with shaking the hand.
- **Anatomy Involved:** The median nerve traverses the carpal tunnel in the wrist and can be compressed by overuse or inflammation.
- **Clinical Correlates:**
    - Positive Phalen's and Tinel's signs.
    - Thenar muscle atrophy in severe cases.
    - Diagnosis confirmed by nerve conduction studies.
- **Management:**
    - Wrist splinting and NSAIDs for mild cases.
    - Surgical decompression for refractory symptoms.

Case 11: Chronic Shoulder Pain Post-Rotator Cuff Repair

Clinical Presentation: A 55-year-old male presents with persistent shoulder pain six months after undergoing rotator cuff repair. He reports difficulty lifting objects and performing overhead activities, along with limited range of motion.

Relevant Anatomy:
- The rotator cuff includes the **supraspinatus, infraspinatus, teres minor, and subscapularis** muscles, which stabilize the glenohumeral joint.
- Repair failure may involve the greater tuberosity of the humerus or incomplete tendon healing.

Key Features:
- Postoperative imaging (e.g., MRI) reveals incomplete tendon healing or re-tear.
- Physical examination shows weakness in shoulder abduction and external rotation.

Clinical Correlation: Failure to restore proper attachment of the tendon compromises joint stability and function, requiring revision surgery or physical therapy.

Case 12: Saddle Anesthesia In Cauda Equina Syndrome

Clinical Presentation: A 45-year-old woman presents with lower back pain, progressive bilateral lower limb weakness, and urinary incontinence. Neurological examination reveals reduced sensation in the perianal region.

Relevant Anatomy:
- The **cauda equina** consists of nerve roots below the L1-L2 vertebral level, responsible for sensory and motor function in the lower limbs and bladder.

Key Features:
- Imaging (MRI) shows a large central disc herniation compressing the cauda equina.
- Clinical findings include saddle anesthesia, diminished reflexes, and sphincter dysfunction.

Clinical Correlation: Emergency decompression surgery is required to prevent permanent neurological deficits.

Case 13: Foot Drop After Total Hip Replacement

Clinical Presentation: A 65-year-old male develops weakness in dorsiflexion of the foot and numbness along the lateral shin and dorsum of the foot post-surgery.

Relevant Anatomy:
- The **sciatic nerve** and its peroneal division are at risk during hip arthroplasty.
- Entrapment or stretch injury affects motor and sensory functions.

Key Features:
- Physical examination confirms foot drop and sensory deficits in the peroneal nerve distribution.
- Nerve conduction studies indicate neuropraxia or axonotmesis.

Clinical Correlation: Recovery may require bracing and physiotherapy, with severe cases needing surgical decompression.

Case 14: Trigeminal Neuralgia With Atypical Presentation

Clinical Presentation: A 70-year-old woman reports sudden, intense facial pain triggered by chewing and talking, localized to the mandibular region.

Relevant Anatomy:
- The **trigeminal nerve** (CN V) provides sensory innervation to the face.
- Compression of the nerve root by an aberrant vessel often leads to trigeminal neuralgia.

Key Features:
- MRI shows vascular compression at the nerve root entry zone.
- Symptoms are controlled with carbamazepine.

Clinical Correlation: Severe or refractory cases may require microvascular decompression surgery.

Case 15: Radial Nerve Palsy Following Spiral Humerus Fracture

Clinical Presentation: A 30-year-old male presents after a fall on an outstretched arm, resulting in a midshaft humerus fracture. He reports difficulty extending his wrist and fingers.

Relevant Anatomy:
- The **radial nerve** courses through the spiral groove of the humerus and is prone to injury in midshaft fractures.
- It innervates the wrist and finger extensors.

Key Features:
- Wrist drop (inability to extend the wrist).
- Sensory loss over the dorsal aspect of the hand.

Clinical Correlation: Prompt fracture reduction and splinting are essential. Recovery typically occurs over months, but severe cases may require surgical exploration.

Case 16: Inferior Alveolar Nerve Injury During Wisdom Tooth Extraction

Clinical Presentation: A 28-year-old female complains of numbness in her lower lip and chin after the extraction of an impacted third molar.

Relevant Anatomy:
- The **inferior alveolar nerve** runs through the mandibular canal and provides sensation to the lower teeth, lip, and chin.
- Close proximity to the roots of the lower third molars increases injury risk.

Key Features:
- Paresthesia or anesthesia in the distribution of the inferior alveolar nerve.
- Pain or dysesthesia in the affected region.

Clinical Correlation: Management focuses on observation; most cases resolve spontaneously. Persistent symptoms may require neurosurgical consultation.

Case 17: Median Nerve Compression In Carpal Tunnel Syndrome

Clinical Presentation: A 45-year-old office worker reports nocturnal hand numbness, difficulty gripping objects, and thenar eminence atrophy.

Relevant Anatomy:

- The **median nerve** passes through the carpal tunnel along with nine tendons.
- Compression affects sensory and motor functions in the hand.

Key Features:

- Positive Tinel's and Phalen's tests.
- Sensory loss in the thumb, index, middle, and radial half of the ring finger.

Clinical Correlation: Wrist splinting and corticosteroid injections provide initial relief; severe cases may require surgical decompression.

Case 18: Sciatic Nerve Injury Following Intramuscular Injection

Clinical Presentation: A 34-year-old male develops severe posterior thigh pain and foot drop after a gluteal injection.

Relevant Anatomy:
- The **sciatic nerve** runs deep in the gluteal region, vulnerable to injury if injections are placed too medially or inferiorly.

Key Features:
- Weakness in knee flexion and ankle dorsiflexion.
- Sensory loss in the posterior thigh, leg, and foot.

Clinical Correlation: Immediate cessation of offending activity and physiotherapy are crucial. Persistent deficits may require nerve repair.

Case 19: Ulnar Nerve Entrapment At The Elbow

Clinical Presentation: A 50-year-old male presents with numbness in the fourth and fifth fingers and a weak grip.

Relevant Anatomy:
- The **ulnar nerve** traverses the cubital tunnel at the elbow, where it is prone to compression.

Key Features:
- Claw hand deformity.
- Sensory loss in the ulnar distribution.

Clinical Correlation: Conservative management with padding and activity modification is the first line; surgical decompression may be necessary.

Case 20: Axillary Nerve Injury After Shoulder Dislocation

Clinical Presentation: A 22-year-old male experiences shoulder pain and weakness after an anterior shoulder dislocation during a football game.

Relevant Anatomy:
- The **axillary nerve** wraps around the surgical neck of the humerus and innervates the deltoid and teres minor muscles.

Key Features:
- Weakness in shoulder abduction.
- Numbness over the lateral shoulder.

Clinical Correlation: Prompt reduction of the dislocation and physical therapy are essential. Persistent deficits may require electrodiagnostic studies.

Case 21: Superior Gluteal Nerve Injury After Hip Surgery

Clinical Presentation: A 60-year-old female develops a Trendelenburg gait after undergoing hip arthroplasty.

Relevant Anatomy:
- The **superior gluteal nerve** innervates the gluteus medius and minimus muscles, stabilizing the pelvis during walking.

Key Features:
- Positive Trendelenburg sign (pelvic drop on the opposite side).
- Weakness in hip abduction.

Clinical Correlation: Rehabilitation focuses on strengthening the hip abductors. Severe cases may require surgical intervention.

TIPS AND TRICKS FOR APPLIED ANATOMY IN PRACTICE

How To Read Imaging For Anatomical Clues

Interpreting imaging studies is a critical skill for applying anatomical knowledge in clinical practice. The following tips can enhance your ability to identify key anatomical landmarks and abnormalities:

1. **Understand Standard Planes:**
   - **Axial:** Cross-sectional views, often used in CT and MRI scans.
   - **Coronal:** Divides the body into anterior and posterior sections.
   - **Sagittal:** Divides the body into left and right halves.

2. **Start with Normal Anatomy:**
   - Always review normal imaging to familiarize yourself with typical anatomical structures.
   - Use reference atlases or imaging guides for comparison.

3. **Follow a Systematic Approach:**
   - In **head CT scans**, start with the brain, examine the ventricular system, and then check the cranial bones and sinuses.
   - In **chest X-rays**, review the ABCDE

method: Airways, Bones, Cardiac silhouette, Diaphragm, and Everything else.

4. **Identify Symmetry:**
   - Compare structures on both sides of the body to detect abnormalities, such as asymmetrical muscle or organ enlargement.

5. **Look for Common Pathological Signs:**
   - **Spinal X-rays:** Loss of disc height suggests degeneration.
   - **Chest X-rays:** Mediastinal widening could indicate aortic dissection.

6. **Use Contrast Studies for Better Detail:**
   - Intravenous contrast highlights vascular structures and masses.
   - In gastrointestinal imaging, barium studies can delineate the esophagus, stomach, and intestines.

Key Questions To Ask In Trauma And Surgical Cases

To apply anatomical insights effectively in trauma and surgery, consider these essential questions:

1. **What Are the Anatomical Boundaries of the Injury?**
   - Determine which compartments, planes, or cavities are affected.
   - E.g., in abdominal trauma, assess if the injury crosses the peritoneal cavity.

2. **Which Neurovascular Structures Are at Risk?**

- Map out nearby nerves, arteries, and veins that could be compromised.
- E.g., in a midshaft humerus fracture, check for radial nerve injury.

3. **Are There Potential Spaces for Complications?**
   - Know spaces where blood, pus, or air can accumulate, such as the pleural or retroperitoneal spaces.
4. **What Are the Surgical Landmarks?**
   - Be familiar with key landmarks to avoid inadvertent damage.
   - E.g., in hernia repair, recognize the ilioinguinal nerve to prevent entrapment.
5. **What Functional Deficits Might Occur?**
   - Anticipate possible impairments based on the structures involved.
   - E.g., after pelvic trauma, assess for bladder or bowel dysfunction.

Mnemonics And Memory Aids For Anatomy

Effective mnemonics can simplify the memorization of complex anatomical details:

1. **Cranial Nerves (Sensory, Motor, or Both):**
   - Mnemonic: **"Some Say Marry Money, But My Brother Says Big Brains Matter More."**
   - Corresponds to the sensory (S), motor (M), or both (B) functions of cranial nerves I–XII.
2. **Branches of the External Carotid Artery:**
   - Mnemonic: **"Some Angry Ladies Fight Off PMS."**
     - S: Superior thyroid artery

- A: Ascending pharyngeal artery
- L: Lingual artery
- F: Facial artery
- O: Occipital artery
- P: Posterior auricular artery
- M: Maxillary artery
- S: Superficial temporal artery

3. **Carpal Bones (Wrist Bones):**
   - Mnemonic: **"Some Lovers Try Positions That They Can't Handle."**
     - S: Scaphoid
     - L: Lunate
     - T: Triquetrum
     - P: Pisiform
     - T: Trapezium
     - T: Trapezoid
     - C: Capitate
     - H: Hamate

4. **Heart Valves (Flow of Blood):**
   - Mnemonic: **"Try Pulling My Aorta."**
     - T: Tricuspid valve
     - P: Pulmonary valve
     - M: Mitral valve
     - A: Aortic valve

5. **Rotator Cuff Muscles:**
   - Mnemonic: **"SITS."**
     - S: Supraspinatus
     - I: Infraspinatus
     - T: Teres minor
     - S: Subscapularis

6. **Brachial Plexus (Roots, Trunks, Divisions, Cords, Branches):**
    - Mnemonic: **"Randy Travis Drinks Cold Beer."**
        - R: Roots
        - T: Trunks
        - D: Divisions
        - C: Cords
        - B: Branches
7. **Liver Segments (Portal Vein):**
    - Mnemonic: **"Caudate 1 Always Right 2,3. Left 4a/b."**
        - Helps recall the Couinaud liver segment classification.

Recommended Resources For Advanced Study

1. **Textbooks**
   - **Gray's Anatomy for Students** (Latest Edition): A comprehensive resource for foundational and applied anatomy.
   - **Clinically Oriented Anatomy by Moore and Dalley**: Focuses on clinical relevance and case studies.
   - **Netter's Atlas of Human Anatomy**: A visually rich guide with detailed illustrations.

2. **Atlases and Imaging Resources**
   - **Rohen's Color Atlas of Anatomy**: Features photographic dissections of anatomical structures.
   - **Felson's Principles of Chest Roentgenology**: A practical guide for interpreting chest imaging.
   - **Anatomy.tv by Primal Pictures**: An interactive 3D anatomy platform useful for detailed visualization.

3. **Online Platforms**
   - **Radiopaedia**: A leading resource for radiological anatomy and clinical cases.
   - **AnatomyZone**: Free online videos and tutorials for applied anatomy.
   - **Kenhub**: Offers anatomy quizzes, mnemonics, and videos tailored for healthcare professionals.

4. **Apps and Mobile Tools**
   - **Complete Anatomy by 3D4Medical**: A

detailed 3D anatomy learning platform.
- **Muscle Premium**: Focuses on musculoskeletal anatomy for clinical practice.
- **Essential Anatomy 5**: A mobile resource ideal for on-the-go learning.

5. **Peer-reviewed Journals and Articles**
   - **Clinical Anatomy**: Focuses on the application of anatomy in clinical practice.
   - **The Journal of Anatomy**: Covers the latest research in anatomical sciences.
   - **Surgical and Radiologic Anatomy**: Integrates imaging and anatomical studies with surgical relevance.

ABOUT THE AUTHOR

Dr Essam Abdelhakim

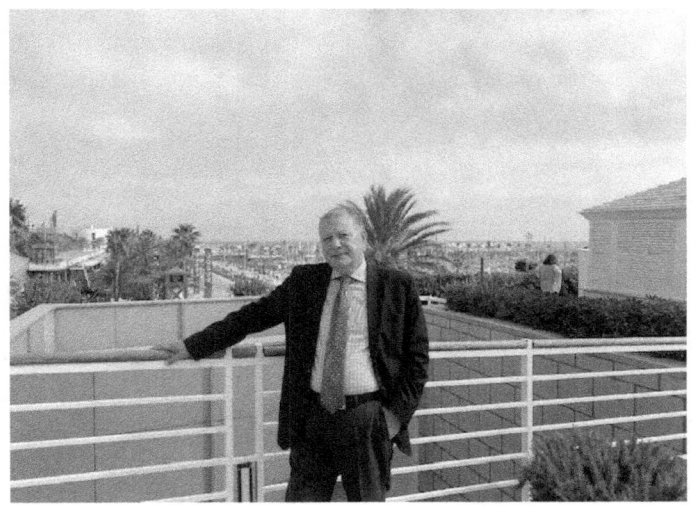

Senior Consultant and Expert in Medical Education

www.ingramcontent.com/pod-product-compliance
Lightning Source LLC
Chambersburg PA
CBHW070405230526
45471CB00006B/2680